YOU AGAIN?

"The story of my second battle with cancer."

Table of Contents

PROLOGUE

The story I am about to relay to you is frustrating, sad, scary, and a bit terrifying. I want to be very clear that I am in no way blaming my caregivers for anything. I just want to positively redirect my patient experience into a learning path for patients and physicians about the advocation of self and communication. They are all excellent and intelligent individuals. I think that overall, it is difficult for people to imagine that there is something actually wrong with me because of my normally fierce status and the amount of people who rely on me on any given day. I get that. I think the other thing that I hear is that I do not "stomp and scream enough." Now my thinking on that what is supposed to be a compliment is that if I had the energy to stomp and scream, I probably wouldn't be as sick. Just sayin.

INTRODUCTION

Hey guys, it's Dr. Katz again. Some of you may remember me from my first cancer book OK It's My Turn Now from a couple of years ago. That described my battle with Hodgkin's Lymphoma, the "good kind" of cancer. Well, now my latest surprise for 2023/2024 is that I have a different kind of "good cancer." It is a diffuse large b cell primary CNS lymphoma of my brain. This is usually reserved for HIV-positive patients. Well, thank God my HIV has been negative multiple times so at least no additional surprise there.

So, that's two different cancers in three years. My stem cells have got to have gotten screwed up somehow so I will be looking forward to stem cell treatment WHEN (not IF dangit) I achieve remission.

So, now that I have brought you up to date, let's get on with this scary, frustrating, and fascinating story.

Dedication

I would like to dedicate this book to my amazing army. You all know who you are and I would not be here today without you.

Also I like to dedicate this book to my amazing team of intelligent and kind physicians. I know that I gave you a run for your money and I was unexpected in multiple ways. I want to say how much I appreciate your knowledge and your thoughtful plans for my care. You are part of the reason that I was able to live and write this book. I hope this can be a part of a pathway to continuing patient care excellence and the survival of more patients to be able to continue to contribute to the world.

I want to encourage the physicians of the world to embrace and celebrate the educated and interested patient. It is absolutely an essential blessing to care for someone so willing to be involved in their own care and be a part of their own solution.

CHAPTER 1: BUT I KEEP TELLING YOU I CAN'T SEE! ISN'T THAT A PROBLEM?

So, back in July of 2023, I started having vision problems consisting of weird flashing lights in the periphery of my vision followed by floaters. I get it that I am getting older, but it still felt like something was wrong with me because I had never had those symptoms before. So I dutifully went to the eye doctor multiple times and they examined me thoroughly and couldn't really find anything. Figuring that they were the experts I kept following up and following up. We won't say how many times. Then, the symptoms progressed to me not being able to see in the dark anymore and then eventually days of complete loss of vision. Now I was terrified. On top of that, I found myself randomly off balance at times. I was cracking my head or my butt with my falls. I went back to the eye doctor and said something was wrong. We need to look harder. I want to see the retinal specialist. Fortunately, I got in right away (which is a relative term after the big delay already) and got some additional pictures and studies. There were some weird changes suggestive of a possible posterior vitreous detachment and uveitis. I was given steroid injections in my eyes which almost immediately restored my daytime vision but did not really address the floaters and flashing lights. I asked about a referral elsewhere because I really felt that something was wrong. I ended up getting referred outside of town and at the very first visit, the doctor told me that I probably had cns lymphoma. OMG! What?! I mean you think the worst and you were trying to get it solved and you knew you weren't done with getting answers but whaaaat?! Cancer again? In my brain? This clean livin is getting me nowhere...lol Now what do we do?

CHAPTER 2: NOW WHAT DO WE DO?

Well, I need to back up for a minute. The first visit to the out-of-town doctor was a bust. We drove all the way there just to be told after we were already there that they couldn't do an accurate exam on me because I had just gotten steroids. This was, to say the least, frustrating and disappointing and it meant delaying seeing them for another month. To be fair the immediate problem of loss of vision was solved enough to function so we proceeded to wait and went back in a month. That was a scary couple of weeks of anticipation. I have to admit at the time that I was already thinking that just the steroids were not going to obscure visualization of what was going on in my head, but we followed the expert's advice. I just had a simmering fear in my head that any additional waiting was not going to be good.

CHAPTER 3: BACK TO THE UVEITIS SPECIALIST

We finally made it back to the uveitis specialist. In the meantime, my vision was still semi-hanging in there at least during the daytime so I could still function. Nighttime was still terrible. I could not see in the dark and was stumbling around. I finally met the uveitis specialist, and she concluded from the previous pics from my ophthalmologist and the retinal specialist that it looked like a cns lymphoma from the changes she saw. What?! Was nobody else going to mention this? How much difference or advancement has this month made? I found myself starting to panic a bit. Now we needed to hurry up and get an MRI of my brain. Nobody could fit me in for weeks anywhere we tried to get in. I knew things were getting worse and I was scared. Fortunately, I had a routine appointment with my endocrinologist who wisely pointed me in the direction of a local independent site MRI and radiology center and I was able to get in right away. Thank the lord for their timeliness. Now the story from here is surprisingly muddled in my brain and has been the victim of subsequent significant short-term memory loss. So, I am relying on what others have told me for this part of the story.

CHAPTER 4: ON TO NEUROSURGERY

Surprise there were a bunch of dragon-shaped tumors and swelling in my brain. This prompted a visit to a neurooncologist and a referral to a different specialty center. We were also referred for a very necessary brain biopsy to be performed by a neurosurgeon at yet another hospital. Even this process was not progressing fast enough for me. It still wasn't until December that we were able to get in for this brain biopsy. Again, the details are fuzzy for me because I was apparently already suffering from decreased function and short-term memory issues. I am told that I had just performed a significant amount of successful and difficult surgical procedures days before my brain surgery. My husband and I were wandering around killing time before preop check-in. At that point, I still knew who and where I was. Just a mere few hours later as my husband was helping me to check in for surgery, I didn't know my name or birth date. They helped me check in anyway. My husband was very scared and wanted to take me to the ER instead. By an amazing twist of fate, the neurosurgeon was rounding through at the same time and encouraged him to keep me in the preop area because this procedure had to be done, and an ER visit would have just prolonged things even more in this life-threatening decompensating situation. The story from here is completely dependent on input from others so I will relay what I can. I am told that I successfully underwent brain surgery and was coming out of anesthesia. I looked at my husband and said hi and then became encephalopathic, turned over, and went into a coma for days. Repeat scans and a stay at the neuro ICU, none of which I remember, revealed a significant increase in tumor growth and swelling to the point that visualization of normal brain tissue was almost impossible. I was also showing seizure activity on my eeg testing but no outward seizure symptoms. In other words, I consider it a miracle that we made it to the right place at the right time so that my life could be saved because things had progressed so far. I was told later that no one could believe that I was even still standing on two feet.

I am grateful to report that they were able to stabilize me with seizure meds and steroids and extensive monitoring. I am also told that my husband stayed by my side for all of those days and sang to me and held my hand while declaring to the nurses and doctors that my brain was the most fierce and brilliant brain he had ever known, and it was imperative that it be saved. I can't even imagine what he was going through watching me disappear right in front of his face, not knowing if I would ever come back. He truly is my life partner, my best friend, my lover, my hero, and the man I am meant to be with forever.

Eventually, I came out of my coma with a silly grin on my face and demonstrated some mental deficits and picking and biting behavior. Apparently, I was trying to chew on my husband and pick at my brain surgery stitches at the same time. Fortunately, I stopped doing that eventually...lol After multiple days I was felt to be well enough to be out of the neuro ICU and then transferred to a step-down unit and then transferred to rehab at yet another hospital. Apparently, my children visited me, but I have no memory of this. It was like being erased.

CHAPTER 5: NOW IT'S TIME FOR REHAB.

The first concrete memories that I have are waking up at the rehab hospital, wondering what the hell was going on, and having things re-explained to me. I am not sure how no one seemed to realize that I was not taking in anything that was going on before that. Anyway, I worked really hard at rehab to get mobile again. Got a bunch of scans that at least had the decency to show that my previous cancer from 2 plus years ago was still gone and it was "just" the brain cancer that was still present. Oh, just brain cancer.

CHAPTER 6: LET'S GET THAT TREATMENT GOING. IT'S DECEMBER ALREADY!

After I finished rehab and my conscious state and functioning continued to improve, (thank God for steroids reducing my cerebral edema) it was time to transfer me to another tertiary center to get my chemo port placed. Treatment had already started using PICC lines. Yuck! Picc lines are the worst in my opinion. They hurt. They bruise. You can't really use your arm. The port is definitely the way to go. We are already in January now. I finally got my port placed on January 3rd after my first treatment. I then got put on a week's chemo schedule for the next two months. One week of 4-day inpatient therapy with methotrexate and rintuximab and one session of outpatient rintuximab in the alternate week. In the midst of all that was oral chemo with temadar as well. Sheesh enough already!

I have to admit, that this schedule is pretty intense and lonely at times. Being in the hospital by yourself for 5 days at a time is a pretty lonely experience. Most of the hospital time is spent trying to clear the rest of the methotrexate out of your system to the point that you are not toxic to the people around you. I never knew that. You learn something new every day.... when your brain is finally working again.

CHAPTER 7: YOU ARE MIRACULOUS!

The good news is that I had a repeat MRI after only two cycles and the radiologist used the phrase significant improvement three different times! This was amazing! It is tough to get a good word out of a radiologist. I finally got to look at my scans side by side when I was conscious enough to even realize I was looking at them. Wow! The difference was incredible! The first scan looked like a bunch of mush and edema and a kind of dragon-shaped tumor with wings and the second scan had far less edema and some actual recognizable brain in it! I was thrilled. We were due for our post neurosurgery follow-up. I really wanted to meet my neurosurgeon. I know that sounds silly since technically I had met him several times already, but this would be the first time I would be conscious enough to realize or remember it. I remember that day. They were just going to have me see the PA, but I really wanted to see the surgeon himself. They couldn't understand why until I explained that this would be the first time I would actually remember and register that I saw him. Then, they understood. They said we would have to wait longer, and we firmly asserted that it would be worth it. I wanted to see his face and remember it. I wanted him to see me and all the progress I had made in just two months. I just needed that affirmation, and I wanted to make his day, and I knew he hadn't seen me really since I was unconscious.

I can remember right when he walked in the exam room door that day. He literally stopped and did a double take and actually smiled...behind his mask. My husband insisted that he never smiles. The neurosurgeon literally said oh my god, you are miraculous! What an awesome compliment! I was beaming underneath my mask too! I know that a lot of the credit for my improvement has to go to the drugs and the steroids, but I wanted to believe that my sheer fortitude tenacity, and desire to live had to have helped some. He said he had never seen anybody come back so fast. He actually wanted to hug me, but we bumped elbows instead.... for safety...lol Let's just say it was an

awesome visit. We were literally singing in
the car on the way home.

CHAPTER 8: I THINK THAT THE COMBINATION OF BEING A BADASS AND HAVING A HISTORY OF GETTING RARE STUFF REALLY IS LIKE A DOUBLE-EDGED SWORD.

This is something that occurred to me at 230 am in the middle of chemotherapy so I had to get it off my chest.

So, let's be honest. I have had some rare stuff in my time starting from the heterotopic pregnancy in my 30s to the Hodgkins lymphoma in my 50s instead of my teens or 60s and now the primary CNS lymphoma without being an immunocompromised HIV-positive individual. I admit it, despite the fierce self-advocating that I do, I just don't fit the criteria most of the time.

Adding to the challenging factor of timely diagnosis is also the fact that I truly believe that it is difficult for most people trying to care for me that something could actually be seriously wrong with me. I do not for one-second hold that against them, but it really is my impression that this is the case. I take great pride in how I have cared for and advocated for people my whole life and how I am able to set aside any personal attachments to cloud my judgement about the patient's total picture and condition, regardless of what I wish wasn't happening. Even now while I am in the hospital getting chemo, I am still fielding phone calls and helping others because I can and because every day I get to wake up, open my eyes, and function on my own is a true blessing.

Has anyone actually confessed that they have trouble caring for me? Of course, not and I would not expect them to. I get it. Last time I checked, doctors are human too, and frankly, they are not generally used to cooperative and knowledgeable patients who have pre-researched, are very familiar with their own bodies, and are attempting to hand over diagnoses that they have pre-contemplated. I don't expect them to be. I hold nothing against them. I treasure all of my healthcare givers to this day and will continue to do so. I just want to be able to use my experiences, provided that I get to live, to educate them and use them as lessons to further guide my care for my own patients.

You know, people always tell me that the reason that I am so good at paying attention and communicating with my patients is because I have been through so much stuff. I think that this may have some partial truth to it, but it is mostly baloney. I have always made it my personal mission to do the best job that I can to advocate communicate and advise my patients. I have never been any different. Even though I am "just a gynecologist" I examine and care for the whole patient, not just their hinterlands. I have diagnosed the full spectrum of obgyn issues and cancers in addition to head-to-toe issues of the whole body. If I don't know much beyond how to diagnose something that is not obgyn, you bet your booty that I research it thoroughly so that I can be a part of supporting and educating the patient and advising them through their impending difficult process. That is my beloved and sacred job and is a large part of keeping me going through all this rough stuff I have been going through. I am fully determined not to be done. I have too much left to offer my family, my patients, and myself. You can't get rid of me that easily. I am too determined (and compliant) to turn this thing around. I have too much to fight for.

CHAPTER 9: HOW CAN YOU POSSIBLY THINK OF YOURSELF AS BLESSED? YOU HAVE BRAIN CANCER FOR CHRISSAKE!

I know you are probably wondering, where is she going with this? Well, let me elaborate. As the news of my cancer spread, more and more people would ask me how I am feeling. My usual answer was "I feel blessed every day." This would prompt the strangest and most confused looks anyone could possibly make. What makes you think that I'm not blessed?" The person uniformly would be taken aback and say something like "How in the hell could you feel blessed? You have brain cancer. You almost died already. You had cancer 3 years ago too. Your husband almost died. What is the blessing in that?"

Well, in these situations I would put on my biggest smile and say, "It truly comes down to a matter of perspective and gratitude. "I am blessed because now I am no longer unconscious. I am blessed because I get to open my eyes every day. I am blessed because I get to talk again. I am blessed because I got to travel the path from the brink of death with coma, seizures, encephalopathy, no vision, and no memory to where I am today." I am blessed that I get to talk again. I am blessed that I get to care for my animals. I am blessed that my recovery so far has been nothing short of miraculous." I get it. A lot of terrible crap has gone on and to be honest, my brain cancer had probably gotten farther than it needed to before I was diagnosed. But, nonetheless, I still get to be here. It is all gravy after that. That is probably way more of a detailed answer than they wanted to hear, but that is the truth.

Usually, this leads to a productive conversation on the power of attitude, positivity, and willingness to survive and the impact of each of those qualities on your personal path through cancer. I cannot emphasize enough the impact of a positive attitude in a cancer battle. Yes. It really is a battle for your life. The drugs and treatments are brutal but magnificent at the time. However, they do not push you into remission all by themselves. You have to play a part. No part of you or your body can afford the energy drain that negativity brings. I am not talking about ignoring the facts of your situation. They are in fact awful. But, you are not doing yourself any favors by getting all down about it. Don't get me wrong, I probably have a cry at least once a week due to something or other just because I hit my tipping point for the week. But I don't let that turn into an overflowing wave of negativity. There is just no point to it. It won't get you cured any faster. You have to stay strong. You have to follow the recommendations. You have to maintain some aspects of positivity. You have to believe that there is a chance you will be cured. You have to be the captain of your own team. You cannot give up before you even begin. In a three-month time period, I progressed from an unconscious state, responsive to painful stimuli only, falling all the time and losing my vision to acting like myself again. I....am.... blessed...and I worked my ass off too!

CHAPTER 10: OMG I AM ABOUT TO START MY LAST CHEMO! I CAN'T BELIEVE THAT TIME HAS COME ALREADY!

Here we are months into the process. Lots and lots of chemo. Lots of lonely weeks in the hospital at a time. Yes, this time the majority of chemo was inpatient. This time I was receiving rintuximab and methotrexate in iv form and temadar orally. They are all devils but very effective in their own rights. The side effect lists are enormous and knowing me, I got some of them, especially the gi ones. Yikes those meds gave the term "ass of fire" a whole new significance for me...lol.

Why inpatient chemo you ask? Because the majority of the time, depending on the health of the patient, chemo is outpatient. It's actually much nicer and you get to just go home after a couple of hours instead of spending a week in the hospital. Well with methotrexate that is a definite no-go. At first, I was like methotrexate. What do I need that for? My only previous experience with methotrexate was to use it in small doses to treat tubal pregnancy that did not require surgery.

So, what does it do and why do we need it for my brain? It is an immunosuppressant. It inhibits dihydrofolate reductase and inhibits lymphocyte proliferation. Heh? English, please. OK. So it blocks folate acid production and breaks down rapidly dividing cells (aka tumor cells and other things) and it stops lymphocytes from multiplying rapidly. OOOh, I get it now. The data on methotrexate is phenomenal with lymphomas. The trick is that it is so toxic, that after leaving it in your system for 24 to 48 hours, you have to spend the next three days trying to clear it because apparently, you will be poisonous to everyone around you if you don't. Yikes.

So, now months and months go by. I spend about a week or so in the hospital every other week. Thank goodness after 6 cycles I no longer had to get additional rintuximab so I would get the week off between chemo sessions. This sounds like a great time off but actually the side effects from chemo tend to be cumulative so even if you are not getting it at the time, the side effects still come for days after. But at least you get to be in your own bed, and you get to have access to your own bathtub, because sometimes that is the only thing that will help heal your fire butt from all the diarrhea.

So, now I am almost at the end of the initial inpatient chemo. This is a very tantalizing and exciting thought. Now we have the stays down to 4 days instead. It's all good news. I want to be excited and celebrate....and I'm going to. But the fact of the matter is that I am not done yet.

What do I mean? Well, there is still more to come, but it is my choice to proceed. I have had two different lymphomas in different parts of my body in three years. There has got to be some stem cell screw-up that needs to be corrected. I say let's give it a tweak if there is even a chance of getting me more time off from cancer. I have been teased with 30 years of freedom as a possibility. I am trying not to view that as a promise, but it sure sounds good.

So, what is stem cell therapy? Basically, you get a catheter put into your large veins for meds and chemo, etc. and you get your bone marrow aspirated down to nothing. Hopefully, I will be asleep for this because it sounds painful. Your bone marrow is a spongy substance in the center of the bones. It produces bone marrow stem cells. Bone marrow stem cells are red blood cells, white blood cells, and platelets. There are also embryonic stem cells that become brain, heart, muscle, bone cells, etc. No other cells in the body have the power and natural ability to generate new cell types. That is pretty fascinating. I am very lucky. It looks like I will qualify for an autologous stem cell transplant. That means that we can use our own cells instead of looking for a donor and worrying about rejection possibilities.

So, what are the general steps? The first is tests and exams. I have had blood work, cardiac echo, and pulmonary function tests. MRI, dental checks, covid tests to assess my overall health. Then,there is the harvesting stage where stem cells are collected in this case from me as an autologous donor. They basically empty you to the point of near death. Your counts will be low to non-existent. You will feel like crap. Then there is conditioning with high dose chemo treatment to prepare you for the transplant. Then there is the transplant part itself and then the recovery period. Most data says that once your counts reach 30 percent or so of normal levels you can go home to complete recovery. This still means several weeks in the hospital either way. I know what you're thinking. Isn't it safer to actually stay in the hospital until your counts are all the way back up? Actually no. It's a scary thought for my family because they will have to basically put me in a bubble with 24-hour assistance when I get home. There are all kinds of changes we have to make before I could go home anyway. Those are the topics for the upcoming family meeting. Oh boy.

CHAPTER 11: THE LAST INITIALLY SCHEDULED INPATIENT CHEMO IS DONE!

The moment I realized that those last drops went in, and my kidneys cleared out enough methotrexate to actually go home, I felt like I should have heard the trumpets sounding, got to ring the bell, and started to party. Right? Well, actually I was just exhausted, a little tearful, and ready to go home. I really couldn't process anything else at the moment. My body and my mind had kind of had it at that point. I just wanted to go home and stay there for more than a few days. All these months were pretty lonely times. Whole weeks at the hospital, months even in the beginning. It's a lot. Compared to my previous cancer, which was all outpatient chemo, this was a lot tougher. It was a strange process. I would spend a lot of time getting psyched up to go to the hospital, telling myself I was getting one step closer to done, and yet, I would still have my weekly cry out of steroid bursts and out of nowhere and would just be exhausted by the time it was time to go home. The recoup time got longer each time also. That is understandable though. Those chemo devils like to be accumulative in terms of side effects. The weird thing is that a part of me actually got excited about the intensifying side effects because what they actually meant is that I had a more viable brain for the drugs to get to. How's that for a fine how do you do...lol. So, there were no parades or fanfare. I just got to go home. Still good though.

CHAPTER 12: BRING ON THE STEM CELL!

Ok so just when you think you are done...you're not! You start thinking "Sweet! Chemo is done! Bye hospital." You get a little cocky and start fantasizing about the journey being over and ...wait a minute....it hits you. You have had two totally different lymphomas within three years. Something is screwy in the baseline. Is this the pace I have to look forward to? Cancer every two to three years? Time off work. Risk of dying? Risk of my business dying that I have built over 25 years? Risk of never seeing my family or friends or doing anything normal consistently?

I thought to myself, there has to be something I can do to tweak this baseline foolishness. I am not saying I wouldn't keep up that pace if I had to, because I am fully committed to remaining on the planet and putting love out there and helping my family and patients, but who wants to to tell you the truth?

Well, there is something that I could do. I could do stem cell therapy. For the first time in all my cancer journeys thus far, I was the perfect candidate for something. It was particularly good for my type of lymphomas. I could donate cells to myself which cuts down on all of the reaction and graft failure risks. And...my risk of mortality at the facility of my choosing was less than 1%. Well shit, my risk of being hit by a car or any of these cancers killing me already is higher than that when I think about it. I'm thinkin let's give it a whirl. The first part of all of this was not my choice, but this part could be.

CHAPTER 13: I HAD A BENEFIT!

Yep, it's true. People that cared about me threw me a benefit. I couldn't believe it! They were holding it during my prime nap time, so I was nervous. But, I actually stayed awake the whole time! We actually raised a significant amount of money, which is already all gone due to medical bills but lord it helped so much. We served amazing homemade food. I had all kinds of volunteers. We had volunteer performers including my daughters and husband. It was awesome! I was so touched. I was super worried about people being offended that I couldn't hug them, but my peeps created a no-hug zone, and I masked up for safety and everyone seemed ok with it. Whew. I just didn't want to offend anybody or make them think I didn't appreciate every last thing they did for me. I would and have done anything for them also. I guess I didn't need to worry.

You know what was really great? Everybody in that room had a story about how I had helped them or saved their life. Awesome! They were unsolicited stories. They just were people wanting to be there and support and share positive info. I was so so grateful. To be honest, I don't do anything with the goal of praise. I do it because it is my life's mission to help people and empower women and patients until I can't any longer. Still, it is pretty wonderful to realize what an impact you are actually making.

CHAPTER 14: IT'S TIME FOR THE STEM CELL EXTRACTION!

What the heck is a stem cell extraction? Let me explain. The stem cell extraction or harvest is the process that is used to prepare for a future stem cell transplant. Ok, let's back up even further. Why the heck am I getting a stem cell transplant and what the heck is it supposed to do? Don't I want to be done already?

The simple answer is yes, I would love to be done already. The reality is that I am really not done already because I have had two different lymphomas within a three-year time period. I have responded well to chemo both times and looks like I am on track to beat this one too...yay! However, that much cancer in that short amount of time off in between means that there is a baseline stem cell issue that needs to be tweaked. I am actually choosing this path to help me get a little more time off in between, if not permanently off.

So, what is the stem cell transplant process really like? It is a grueling thing with potential amazing rewards, so I have decided to go for it if there is even a slight chance that I won't have to keep up this vicious pace anymore.

Here's how it goes. First, you need to start some stingy painful subcutaneous injections in your abdominal fat for five days before your retrieval. These injections are filled with granulocyte colony-stimulating
factor. What? Heh? This medicine is to literally help you create your own army of stem cells and lymphocytes from within. It is literally charging up your bone marrow to turn a couple of thousand lymphocytes into 50,000 or more. Then, when you get to your last day of these injections you get to report to the hospital for your final injection that begins slamming all these newly created army cells into your peripheral bloodstream so they can be harvested the next day.

As you can imagine, it is pretty hard work creating your own army, with help, from within. Man! The muscle pain and the bone pain are pretty intense and until the Tylenol kicks in, you are kind of limping around like an 80-plus-year-old. Yes, I was offered stronger medicine for pain, but I did not want it. If I could get through the pain with the Tylenol without causing extreme constipation from narcotics I was going to try it.

Now the day of stem cell harvesting has arrived. I have been thoroughly educated and pre-prompted to expect 8 hours of being attached to a space-age-looking plasmapheresis machine for up to 8 hours without even being able to get up to go to the bathroom unless I used a bedpan. Needless to say, I tried to actually minimize my drinking and get my bm out of the way to try to avoid that...lol. No way am I poopin in a bedpan. I get it. The pheresis machine is very sensitive and the slightest move the wrong way and it could stop the whole process. Time to suck it up I guess,

So, we got to the stem cell clinic a few minutes late because our smarty pants selves decided to park right outside the door to the clinic without realizing that this particular door required a badge to get in...oops! We thought we finally had it right. Thank goodness a very nice lady was coming into work and was nice enough to let us in. There is quite a strict time schedule, so we did not want to be late.

So, we arrived and got all hooked up to my newly placed central line triple lumen catheter in my chest. We drew some initial labs to see where we were starting from as far as electrolytes and the number of wbcs and cd34 cells that I had achieved with all the shots. There were certain goals that needed to be achieved to give me a greater chance of getting the whole retrieval done in a single day. Well, guess what? I shot way past the WBC and cd34 goals and they even put in my lab report that I was likely to finish in one day in a single retrieval. The goal was to be able to retrieve 3 million stem cells.

It was true! Not only did I retrieve above and beyond the number of cells to start with, but I actually was able to get 8 million stem cells retrieved in half the normal time. They told me they thought I had sent a record! Awesome! Amazing what following the instructions to the letter can do. They were so kind and flattering. They called me a rock star. That was a great thing to hear. Now it was time to go home and fall into bed and recover for 9 days or so until the admission for the total marrow ablating chemo that was coming.

CHAPTER 15: TIME FOR THE CANNONBALL CHEMO

So, here we are 9 days later. Ready to be admitted for a full month of fun for a stem cell transplant. First, there will be 8 straight days of myelo-ablating chemotherapy to shoot all my counts down to nothing. They are even giving me extra because they think I can handle it. I say yikes, easy on the compliments.

Then I get a day of rest. And then it's on to replacing my stem cells with my harvested cells and hoping that they take in a timely manner. Likely it will take two more weeks or so, so I am still looking at about a month in the hospital. We will see how it goes.

CHAPTER 16: ONLY THREE DAYS LEFT OF PRE-STEM CELL TRANSPLANT CHEMO

So far, I have had three days of thiotepa at high doses. Thiotepa is a beast worthy of respect. It is a very strong alkylating agent. This means that it goes into your body and links DNA strands which then stop DNA, RNA, and protein synthesis, resulting in cell death. It is actually a nitrogen mustard gas derivative, something previously used in chemical warfare. It has come a long way since being modified as an anticancer agent. It has a list of side effects a mile long and can potentially destroy your skin if even a tiny amount is allowed to sit on the skin's surface. So, you end up not being able to use traditional dressings because they may trap the medicine against your skin. You also have to shower, with no soap, every 4 to 6 hours to rinse off any residual medicine. It can also cause incredible mucositis or breakdown of all mucous membranes, especially in the mouth so you must chew ice the entire time the 4-hour infusion is going. Needless to say, I followed those instructions to the letter and thank goodness no skin breakdown or mucositis yet...Whew!

Now we move on to three days of busulfan, also a powerful alkylating agent that alkylates and crosslinks DNA to cause cell death. Again, the list of side effects that are possible is a mile long. My personal favorite thing that I experienced was chest pain. Nothing like being plugged up to chemo, thinking you could be having a heart attack, but you're not. Thank goodness that feeling went away after the infusion was over.

Next comes two days of cyclophosphamide, also an alkylating agent and nitrogen mustard derivative designed to crosslink and alkylate DNA to cause cell death. Surprise surprise it also has a list of side effects a mile long. Here goes nothing.

While I am trying to take it as a compliment that they are giving me extra chemo as a reward for my toughness, it is still somewhat daunting at the same time. It also means I will probably have to be in the hospital longer, which feels like forever when you just want to get back to your own bed and your own house and your family and friends. But, as I have moments of despair or discouragement, I need to keep a healthy mindset and remember that I chose this part to at least give me the chance at more time off cancer and a fuller life.

CHAPTER 17: THE PRETRANSPLANT CHEMO IS DONE. NOW ON TO THE TRANSPLANT

So, I just finished 8 straight days of some of the most brutal myeloid-ablating chemo on the planet. 8 straight days. I hear that most people only due 5 days and only do two kinds of chemo. Well lucky me. They had a lot of confidence in my

toughness and gave me 8 straight days and three different kinds of chemo. Umm, thanks but no thanks at the same time...lol So, I got 8 straight days of some of the toughest chemo on the planet. I mean these are the big kahunas, specifically given with the intent to knock you down to zero...literally. No white blood cells, red blood cells, or platelets for you, my little friend. The kind of side effects and possible organ damage that you can possibly get are almost too intense to pre-read about. But you know me, I wanted to be informed so I read anyway.

I got Thio Tepa, Busulfan, and Cytoxan. These are all crazy-duty heavy alkylating agents. This means that they get right in there and cross-link DNA and destroy cells. Whoo and yikes. Some of them are so bad for your skin that you have to shower every 4 to 6 hours to make sure not even one drop gets on you. Thankfully I followed everything to the painful letter so that didn't happen. The things are that while you are slogging through it you think you are getting away with it when in fact the side effects are still coming.... days after the chemo is over. Surprise!

So now the 8 days of chemo are over, and you get a day of rest before the transplant. At first, I was like who needs to rest? Let's get going. No. No. They know what they are talking about. Suddenly you are all wiped out and really could use a day of rest.

So, you take your day and then transplant day comes. You are all psyched up. They come in with all the machines and gadgets. They come in with over 8 million stem cells you donated for yourself to put back. There are multiple huge bags. Then a ton of people come in to monitor you and record the process. OK. You are ready. Let's go.

Well, I gotta tell ya, for the hours it took to harvest the cells, it only took about 23 min to put them back. What? Heh? That's it? I don't what I was expecting but I was expecting it to take longer or feel something. Nope. It was done before you knew it.

CHAPTER 18: NOW, HURRY UP AND WAIT.

Now the transplant is over, and it is time to wait for the stem cells to re-cooperate, which often takes weeks. You have yourself thinking I'm almost done. I'm almost to the finish line! You are, in a sense. But there will be several weeks left. Time to start walking to make the bone marrow take quicker.

Most research says that if you move enough, you can literally speed up your own process. I was ready to move. I was out there putting in 10000 plus steps a day. I was serious about getting out of there as soon as I could. I just put my earbuds in and went to town. It was a good distractor from how I was feeling. I am not sure how I was able to truck around that much with my hemoglobin and platelets and wbcs in the toilet but I was committed!

Unfortunately, all the self-progress would come to a halt because I got a couple of infections that did not allow me to walk in the hallway. I took this pretty hard because it felt like the one thing, I could do for myself to contribute to getting better. Oh well, room time it was. I still had my peddler in my room, but it wasn't the same as rockin it out to ACDC while tooling around the halls with my husband trying to catch up. Oh well, I made the best of it but kind of felt like a prisoner. I admit it. I had a mini temper tantrum when they stopped me in the hall and made me go back to my room. It was just kind of an icing on the cake with everything else going on. But I made it through. More time to rest and write, I guess.

CHAPTER 19: A KICK IN THE BUTT.

The doctors came in to say that I can go home soon, maybe within days. I was so excited. I can't wait to go home. It's been so long since I've been at home that I start to lose patience a bit at times. I think that is understandable though. Who is ok with spending as much time in the hospital as I have in the last six months? It's some lonely and frustrating business while you are in the hospital fighting for life and your family is fighting to try to get along without you. It's a lot of pressure.

So, I am all excited about the thought of going home. The doc said it might even be the weekend (it's Thursday at the time of this talk so we are still close). But then, it all came down crashing for me when she said she doesn't think they even due discharges on the weekend because the team doesn't like it because they don't feel it's safe. In a few seconds I felt like my hopes were shattered in a single minute. I just wish she hadn't put the idea of an earlier discharge into my head. Now I couldn't stop thinking about that. Of course that's my issue, not the doctors. They didn't mean to do anything wrong. It still set me back a minute, so I had to regain perspective and remind myself that even a few days was not that crucial.

CHAPTER 20: OMG I GET TO GO HOME IN A MATTER OF DAYS!

It's finally happening. The thought of going home is becoming a reality. Home! I will get to go home! My own bed will be there. My family will be there. My pets will be there. My flowers will be there. Yessss! So many good things to look forward to.

I know that my family is excited and worried about me going home. I totally get it. There is a ton to watch for still. There will still be meds and stuff to do. There are a ton of precautions and restrictions. But so, what! Mom will get to be at home! Isn't that the main goal at the end of the tunnel? Feels like it to me. I am reassuring them that there is no capriciousness or rushing going on here. Everything is well throughout, and they are even doing my discharge stuff early so I can just leave when I get to leave. They are bending over backwards for us. I love it. I deserve it. I have put in some of the toughest work of my life toward the goal of spending more time off of cancer. I want the reward. I want to go home.

CHAPTER 21: IT'S TODAY IT'S TODAY!

Omg we are finally here! Discharge day! Time to go home. Time to see the family. Time to see the house. Time to see the yard. Time to see the pets. All of it. I want all of it. I want the freedom of knowing that this time when I get in the car it's to stare out the window to go somewhere that I actually want to go! I want to go lay in my own bed. I want to pet my pets. I want to hug(safely) my family. I want to stare at my beautiful plants and just take in the glory of the earth and the outside world that I have the privilege of living in.

I cannot wait for my husband to get here. I cannot wait to throw my arms around him...if allowed. I can't wait to get in that car and drive off. Storms or sunshine we are outta here! Let's bring on the next phase of my phoenix transformation. I have always been grateful for everything I have. I have worked and fought hard for everything. Nothing has been given. Still, it is amazing how you start assuming things will always be as they are until they aren't anymore. Well, no more assuming for me! I have always been and forever will be grateful for every single everything in my life. I am very fortunate that my life is rich and plentiful in love, relationships, and peace. Time to start enjoying it again!

CHAPTER 22: THE FIRST FOLLOW-UP VISIT.

I can't believe the day is here. It's time for my first follow-up visit after getting discharged after a stem cell transplant. A follow-up visit. This means I am done with the treatment and the stem cell transplant. This means that my counts were high enough to go home. This means that there will be more days of enjoying the sunshine, riding in the Camaro, enjoying my family, and enjoying my pets. I could not be a luckier girl. Every day of freedom outside of the hospital is like a gift. A gift that I am happy and grateful to receive. There has been a ton of work and suffering to be sure. But, if there is even a chance for more time off cancer, it was so worth it.

CHAPTER 23: MY THOUGHTS AT "THE END"

Actually, it really isn't the end, is it? I am now looking forward to at least a 5-year or a lifetime of follow-ups and tests and check-ups. It all depends on how it goes. That sounds like a lot of tedious stuff, but you know, I am so frickin grateful just to be alive, I will dot every I and cross every t and make every follow-up that I need to. These at least will be scheduled things that I actually get to go home after. There really is no downside.

People ask me all the time how I can ever consider myself a lucky person with everything I have been through. I get it. I have been through two cancers in three years. I have struggled to keep my business afloat. I took care of my husband after his heart attack in between my two cancers. I have gone through near financial ruin. These are all pretty crazy things.

But you know what? I am still here! I have put the work in! I have buckled in and put forth my positive mojo and worked my ass off just to survive and I did! Despite all odds, mishaps, and statistics. I even broke records while doing it! This is amazing and terrible at the same time.

I have learned even more as a physician how to help patients cope with the terrible, how to deliver bad news, and how to help them strategize their way through it.

The point is that I got to stay. Everything else does not fade away over time. That is true. But, I got to stay. That is a huge reward. I get to be reminded of how awesome life on earth can be. I get to be with my family. I get to keep caring for women of all ages. That's why I still consider myself a lucky person.